The Joy of Forest Bathing

© 2024 Lachlan McGregor

ISBN: 978-91-531-2833-5

Green Scene Publishing

The Joy of Forest Bathing

Embracing Nature for Health and Happiness

Lachlan McGregor

Chapter 1:	9
The Healing Power of Nature	9
Connecting with Nature:	9
A Natural Remedy for Stress	9
The Science Behind Forest Bathing	11
Benefits of Spending Time in Nature	13
Cultivating Mindfulness in the Great Outdoors	15
Chapter 2:	18
The Beauty of Trees	18
The Majestic Oak:	18
Symbol of Strength and Resilience	18
The Serene Willow: Finding Peace in Nature	20
The Noble Redwood: Standing Tall and Proud	22
The Sacred Cedar: Embracing Ancient Wisdom	24
Chapter 3: Forest Bathing Techniques	26
Mindful Walking: Finding Joy in Every Step	26
Tree Hugging: Harnessing the Energy of Nature	28
Nature Meditation: Quiet the Mind and Open the Heart	30
Forest Breathing: Inhaling Fresh Air for Health and	

| Happiness | 32 |

Chapter 4: Creating Your Own Nature Sanctuary — 35

- Designing a Sacred Space in Your Backyard — 35
- Bringing the Outdoors Inside: Houseplants for Health — 37
- Nature-Inspired Crafts and DIY Projects — 38
- Planning a Nature Retreat: Connecting with the Wild — 40

Chapter 5: Embracing the Seasons — 43

- Spring Renewal: Awakening Your Senses — 43
- Summer Bliss: Basking in the Warmth of the Sun — 45
- Fall Harvest: Celebrating the Bounty of Nature — 47
- Winter Reflection: Finding Peace in Stillness — 49

Chapter 6: The Joy of Forest Bathing for Health and Happiness — 52

- Healing the Body, Mind, and Spirit with Nature — 52
- The Japanese Practice of Shinrin-Yoku — 53
- The Philosophy Behind Shinrin-Yoku — 54
- Health Benefits of Shinrin-Yoku — 54
- How to Practice Shinrin-Yoku — 55

Cultivating Gratitude for the Gifts of the Earth	57
Embracing the Wisdom of the Forest: Lessons in Resilience and Growth	61
Conclusion: Living a Life in Harmony with Nature	63
Acknowledgments	65
Resources for Further Exploration	67
About the Author	69
The Joy of Forest Bathing	72

Chapter 1:
The Healing Power of Nature

Connecting with Nature:
A Natural Remedy for Stress

Are you feeling stressed, overwhelmed, or just in need of a mental reset? Look no further than the healing power of nature. Connecting with the natural world has been proven to be a powerful remedy for stress and anxiety, offering a sense of peace and tranquility that can rejuvenate both body and mind. In this subchapter, we will explore how spending time in nature, particularly among trees, can bring about a sense of calm and well-being that can enhance your overall health and happiness.

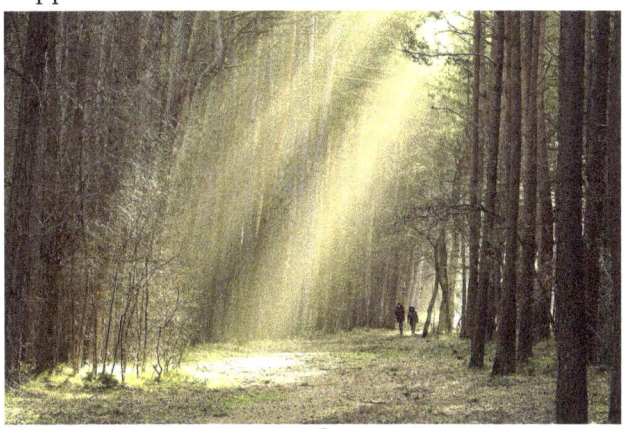

Nature lovers know all too well the transformative power of spending time in the great outdoors. Whether it's taking a leisurely stroll through a forest, sitting beneath the canopy of a majestic tree, or simply breathing in the fresh air, the benefits of connecting with nature are undeniable. Studies have shown that spending time in nature can lower levels of cortisol, the stress hormone, while increasing feelings of happiness and well-being. It's no wonder that so many people turn to nature as a source of comfort and healing in times of stress.

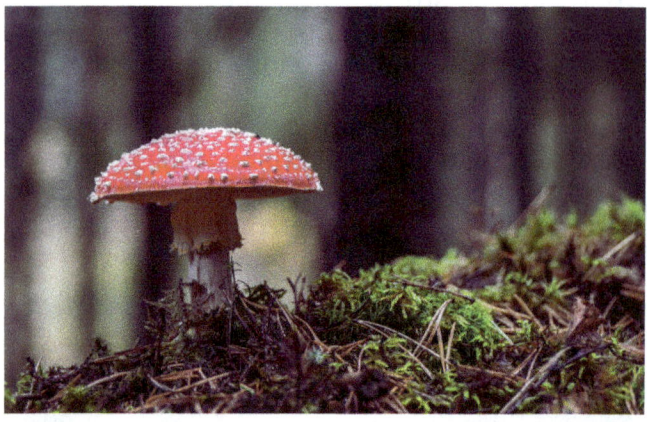

One of the most powerful ways to connect with nature is through the practice of **forest bathing**. Originating in Japan, forest bathing involves immersing oneself in the sights, sounds, and smells of the forest in order to promote relaxation and reduce stress. By mindfully engaging with nature, we can tap into its healing energy and experience a profound sense of connection and peace. The simple act of walking among trees can have a profound impact on our mental and emotional well-being, helping us to feel more grounded, centered, and at peace.

Trees, in particular, have a special ability to soothe our souls and calm our minds. Known as "nature's natural healers," trees emit phytoncides, chemicals that have been shown to boost the immune system and reduce stress. In addition, the presence of trees has been linked to lower levels of anxiety and depression, as well as improved cognitive function and overall well-being. By spending time in the company of trees, we can tap into their restorative powers and experience a sense of peace and harmony that can uplift our spirits and renew our energy.

So next time you're feeling stressed or overwhelmed, consider taking a walk in the woods, sitting beneath a tree, or simply spending time in nature. By connecting with the natural world, you can experience a sense of peace and well-being that can enhance your overall health and happiness.

Embrace the healing power of nature and discover the joy of forest bathing for yourself. Your mind, body, and soul will thank you for it.

The Science Behind Forest Bathing

Welcome to the fascinating world of forest bathing, where science meets nature to create a powerful recipe for health and happiness. In this subchapter, we will explore the science behind forest bathing and how it can positively impact our well-being. Did you know that spending time in nature, particularly among trees, has been scientifically proven to reduce stress and improve overall mental health? The practice of forest bathing, also known as **Shinrin-yoku** in Japan, involves immersing oneself in the sights, sounds, and smells of the forest to reap these incredible benefits. Studies have shown that forest bathing can lower cortisol levels, decrease blood pressure, and boost the immune system, making it a powerful tool for combating the stresses of modern life.

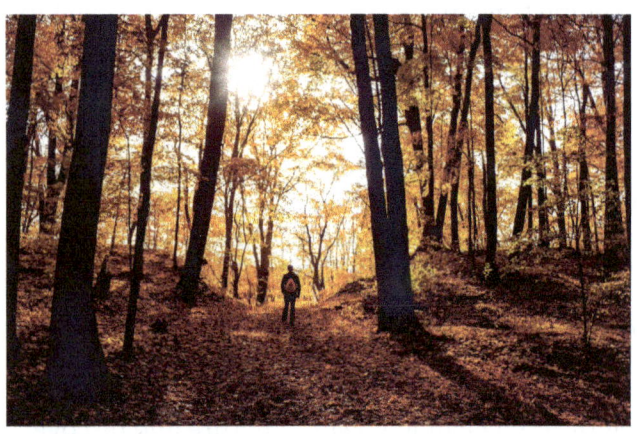

One of the key components of forest bathing is the presence of phytoncides, which are volatile compounds released by trees and plants. These phytoncides have been shown to have anti inflammatory and immune-boosting effects on the body, helping to improve overall health and well-being. Additionally, the sights and sounds of the forest can have a calming effect on the mind, reducing feelings of anxiety and promoting a sense of peace and tranquility.

But the benefits of forest bathing go beyond just physical health – spending time in nature has also been linked to improved creativity, focus, and mood. Studies have shown that being in natural environments can enhance cognitive function and increase feelings of happiness and well-being. So next time you're feeling overwhelmed or stressed, consider taking a walk in the woods to clear your mind and rejuvenate your spirit.

In conclusion, the science behind forest bathing is clear – spending time in nature, particularly among trees, can have a profound impact on our physical and mental health. Head out into the forest, and the healing powers of nature. Your mind, body, and spirit will thank you for it!

Benefits of Spending Time in Nature

Are you a nature lover who feels happiest and healthiest when surrounded by trees and greenery? If so, you're not alone! In this subchapter, we will explore the many benefits of spending time in nature, specifically focusing on how we can get happy and healthy by immersing ourselves in the beauty of the natural world.

One of the key benefits of spending time in nature is the positive impact it has on our mental health. Studies have shown that being in nature can help reduce stress, anxiety, and depression, while also improving mood and overall well-being. The sights, sounds, and smells of the forest can have a calming effect on our minds, allowing us to relax and unwind from the stresses of everyday life.

In addition to its mental health benefits, spending time in nature can also have a positive impact on our physical health. Research has shown that being in nature can help boost our immune system, lower blood pressure, and reduce the risk of chronic diseases such as heart disease and diabetes. The fresh air and clean environment of the forest can help us breathe easier and feel more energized and revitalized.

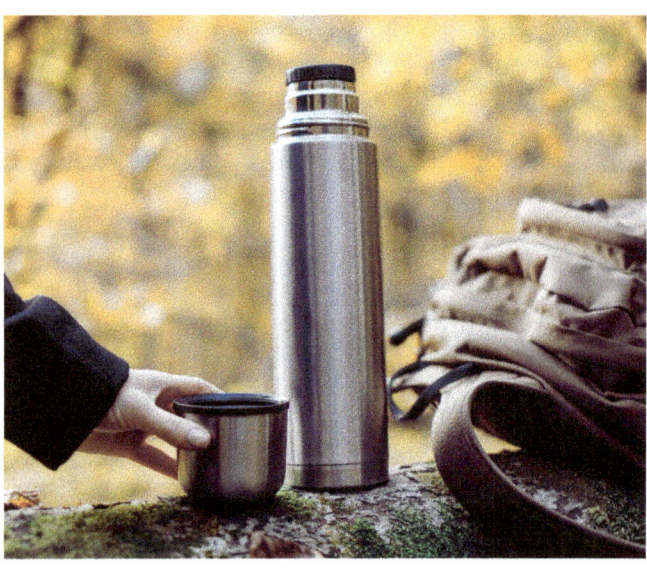

Another benefit of spending time in nature is the opportunity it provides for exercise and physical activity. Whether you're hiking through the woods, cycling along a nature trail, or simply taking a leisurely walk through a park, being in nature encourages us to move our bodies and stay active. This can help improve our fitness levels, strengthen our muscles, and increase our overall physical health.

Furthermore, spending time in nature can also help us connect with others and build strong relationships. Whether we're exploring the forest with friends, family, or a partner, being in nature provides a shared experience that can deepen our connections and strengthen our bonds. The beauty and tranquility of the natural world can inspire meaningful conversations and moments of togetherness that can nurture our relationships and bring us closer to those we care about.

In conclusion, the benefits of spending time in nature are vast and varied, from improving our mental and physical health to enhancing our relationships and overall well-being. So if you're a nature lover looking to get happy and healthy, consider embracing the beauty of the natural world and immersing yourself in the joy of forest bathing. Your mind, body, and spirit will thank you for it!

Cultivating Mindfulness in the Great Outdoors

Are you a nature lover seeking to enhance your health and happiness through the power of the great outdoors? Look no further than the practice of cultivating mindfulness in the great outdoors. In this subchapter, we will explore how immersing yourself in nature can bring about a sense of peace and well-being, and how you can harness the healing benefits of trees and natural surroundings to boost your overall health and happiness.

Spending time in nature has been shown to reduce stress, improve mood, and increase feelings of well-being. By practicing mindfulness in the great outdoors, you can deepen your connection to the natural world and experience a profound sense of calm and tranquility. Whether you're taking a leisurely stroll through a forest, sitting by a babbling brook, or simply basking in the beauty of a sunlit meadow, the benefits of being present in nature are undeniable.

One of the most powerful ways to cultivate mindfulness in the great outdoors is through the practice of forest bathing. This Japanese practice involves immersing yourself in the sights, sounds, and smells of the forest, allowing your senses to awaken to the beauty of the natural world around you. By slowing down and tuning in to the present moment, you can experience a deep sense of connection and rejuvenation that can have lasting effects on your health and wellbeing.

In addition to the mental and emotional benefits of cultivating mindfulness in the great outdoors, spending time in nature has been shown to have numerous physical health benefits as well. From reducing inflammation and boosting the immune system to lowering blood pressure and improving cardiovascular health, the healing powers of nature are truly remarkable. By incorporating regular outdoor activities into your routine, you can enhance your overall health and well-being in ways you never thought possible.

So, whether you're an avid nature lover or simply looking to boost your happiness and health, cultivating mindfulness in the great outdoors is a powerful and transformative practice. By immersing yourself in the beauty of the natural world, you can experience a profound sense of peace, well-being, and connection that will leave you feeling rejuvenated and inspired. Embrace the healing benefits of trees and natural surroundings, and discover the joy of forest bathing for yourself.

Chapter 2:

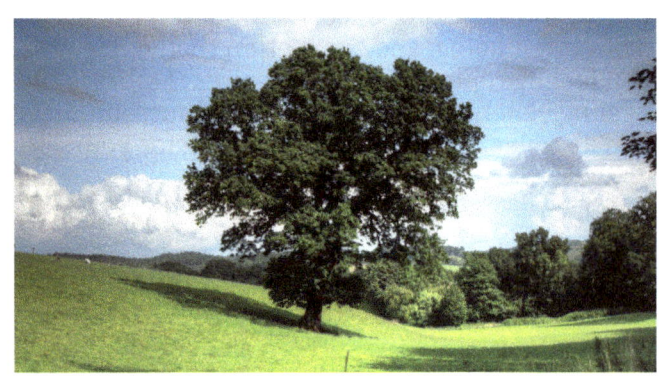

The Beauty of Trees

The Majestic Oak:

Symbol of Strength and Resilience

The majestic oak tree has long been revered as a symbol of strength and resilience in the natural world. Standing tall and proud, with its sprawling branches reaching towards the sky, the oak exudes a sense of power and stability that is truly awe-inspiring. The oak serves as a reminder of the incredible force of nature and the beauty that can be found in even the most rugged landscapes. One of the most remarkable things about the oak tree is its ability to withstand the test of time. Some oak trees can live for hundreds of years, weathering countless storms and changes in the environment without losing their vitality. This resilience is a testament to the tree's incredible strength and adaptability, qualities that we can all aspire to cultivate in our own lives.

In addition to its physical strength, the oak tree is also a powerful symbol of spiritual resilience. In many cultures, the oak is associated with wisdom, courage, and endurance, qualities that are essential for navigating the challenges of life. Spending time in the presence of an oak tree can help to instill a sense of inner strength and resilience, inspiring us to face our own obstacles with grace and determination.

When we immerse ourselves in the presence of the oak tree, we can tap into its energy and draw upon its power to heal and rejuvenate our bodies, minds, and spirits. The practice of forest bathing, or shinrin-yoku, involves spending time in nature and allowing the healing energy of the trees to wash over us, restoring our sense of well-being and vitality. The oak tree, with its strong and grounding presence, is particularly effective at helping us to release stress, anxiety, and negative emotions, leaving us feeling refreshed and renewed.

In conclusion, the majestic oak tree is a powerful symbol of strength and resilience that can inspire and uplift us in our daily lives. By connecting with the wisdom and energy of the oak, we can tap into our own inner reservoirs of strength and endurance, enabling us to face life's challenges with grace and courage. So next time you find yourself in the presence of an oak tree, take a moment to pause, breathe deeply, and allow yourself to be filled with the transformative power of this magnificent tree.

The Serene Willow: Finding Peace in Nature

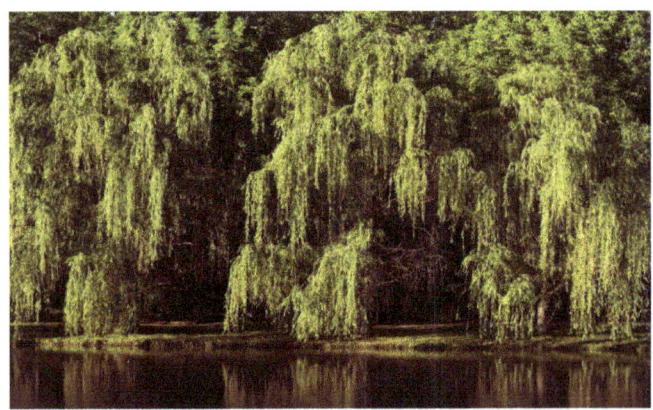

Nature lovers, rejoice! In this subchapter, we will explore the peaceful and calming presence of the serene willow tree and how it can help us find inner peace and tranquility in nature. The willow tree, with its gracefully drooping branches and soft leaves, has long been revered for its calming energy and soothing presence. It is a symbol of strength, flexibility, and resilience, qualities that we can all aspire to embody in our own lives.

When we spend time in the presence of a willow tree, we are enveloped in a sense of peace and harmony that can help us let go of stress, anxiety, and worries. The gentle rustling of the leaves in the breeze, the dappled sunlight filtering through the branches, and the soft, mossy ground beneath our feet all work together to create a serene and tranquil environment that is perfect for relaxation and rejuvenation. Just being near a willow tree can help us feel more grounded, centered, and connected to the natural world around us.

One of the most powerful ways to experience the healing benefits of the serene willow tree is through the practice of forest bathing. Forest bathing, also known as shinrin-yoku in Japan, is the practice of immersing oneself in the sights, sounds, and smells of the forest to promote health and well-being. By taking a leisurely stroll through a forest that is home to willow trees, we can experience the calming effects of nature firsthand and reap the benefits of improved mood, reduced stress, and enhanced overall health.

As we meander through the forest, we can pause to sit beneath a willow tree and meditate, journal, or simply soak in the peaceful energy that surrounds us. We can take deep, cleansing breaths and allow ourselves to be fully present in the moment, letting go of distractions and worries as we connect with the natural world. The serene willow tree acts as a gentle guide, helping us to let go of tension and negativity and embrace a sense of peace and well-being that can stay with us long after we leave the forest.

Next time you find yourself in need of a little peace and tranquility, seek out the serene willow tree and allow yourself to be enveloped in its calming energy. Whether you choose to practice forest bathing, meditate beneath its branches, or simply spend time in its presence, the willow tree can be a powerful ally in your quest for health and happiness. Embrace the healing power of nature and let the serene willow guide you on a journey of peace and rejuvenation.

The Noble Redwood: Standing Tall and Proud

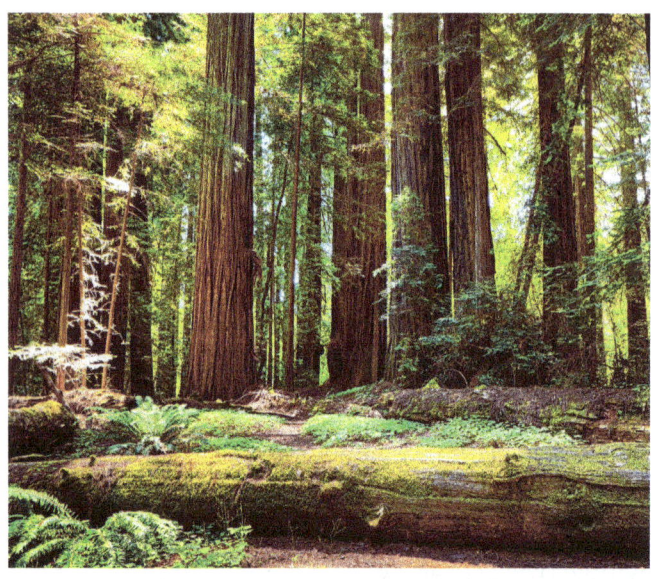

The noble redwood tree, standing tall and proud, is truly a natural wonder to behold. These magnificent giants can reach heights of over 300 feet, making them some of the tallest trees on Earth. Their sheer size and grandeur inspire awe and reverence in all who come across them.The redwood tree represents a symbol of strength, resilience, and beauty in the natural world.

Walking amongst the towering redwoods is a truly transformative experience. The air is crisp and clean, the sunlight filters through the canopy above, and the sounds of nature surround you. Forest bathing, the practice of immersing oneself in the sights, sounds, and smells of the forest, is known to have numerous health benefits. The redwoods, with their serene and majestic presence, provide the perfect setting for this rejuvenating practice.

As you stand at the base of a redwood tree and gaze up at its towering branches, you can't help but feel a sense of peace and tranquility wash over you. The redwoods have a way of grounding us, connecting us to the earth and reminding us of our place in the world. Their presence is a comforting reminder of the beauty and resilience of the natural world, and the importance of preserving and protecting it for future generations.

Many people find solace and healing in the presence of the redwoods. The trees have a way of calming the mind and soothing the soul, helping to reduce stress and anxiety. Studies have shown that spending time in nature, especially amongst trees, can have a positive impact on both our physical and mental well-being. The redwoods, with their ancient wisdom and majestic beauty, offer a sanctuary for those seeking peace and renewal.

In the hustle and bustle of modern life, it is easy to forget the simple joys and healing powers of nature. The redwoods serve as a powerful reminder of the importance of connecting with the natural world and finding moments of peace and serenity amidst the chaos. So next time you find yourself in need of a little pick-me-up, why not take a stroll amongst the redwoods and let their majesty and beauty work their magic on you? Your mind, body, and spirit will thank you for it.

The Sacred Cedar: Embracing Ancient Wisdom

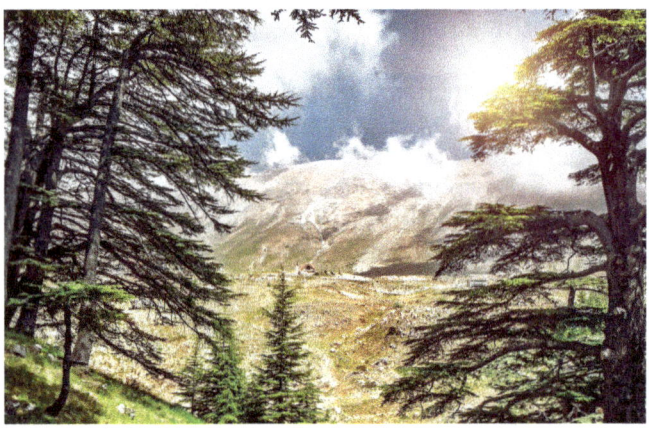

In the heart of the forest, there stands a majestic cedar tree that has witnessed centuries of change and growth. This sacred cedar embodies the ancient wisdom of the forest, offering a sense of peace and tranquility to all who come near.We are drawn to the wisdom and healing powers of trees, and the sacred cedar is a powerful symbol of this connection.

Embracing the ancient wisdom of the sacred cedar is a transformative experience that can bring us closer to nature and ourselves. By spending time in the presence of this wise tree, we can tap into its energy and wisdom, allowing it to guide us on our journey towards health and happiness. The sacred cedar reminds us to slow down, breathe deeply, and connect with the natural world around us.

As we immerse ourselves in the healing powers of the forest, we can feel our stress and worries melt away, replaced by a sense of peace and clarity. The sacred cedar teaches us to let go of our fears and anxieties, and to trust in the wisdom of nature to heal and restore us. By embracing the ancient wisdom of the cedar tree, we can find inner peace and balance in our lives.

The sacred cedar also serves as a reminder of the importance of conservation and reservation of our natural world. As nature lovers, it is our responsibility to protect and honor the sacred trees that have been a source of wisdom and healing for generations. By connecting with the ancient wisdom of the cedar tree, we can deepen our appreciation for the beauty and significance of the natural world.

In conclusion, the sacred cedar is a powerful symbol of the ancient wisdom and healing powers of nature. By embracing this wisdom and connecting with the energy of the forest, we can experience profound healing and happiness. Let us come together to honor and protect the sacred trees that have so much to teach us about the interconnectedness of all living things.

Chapter 3: Forest Bathing Techniques

Mindful Walking: Finding Joy in Every Step

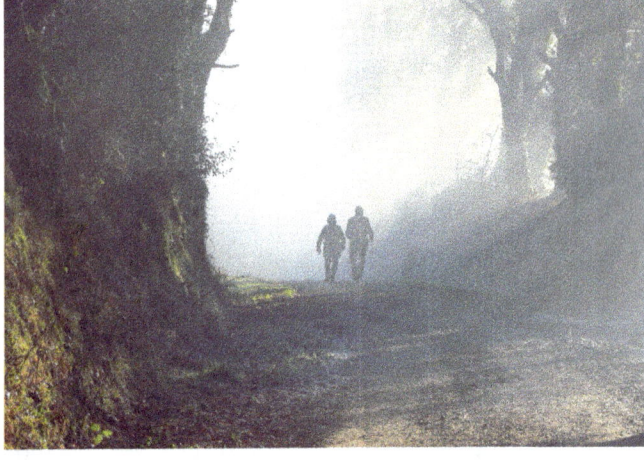

Are you a nature lover who thrives on the beauty of the great outdoors? Do you find yourself rejuvenated and at peace when surrounded by the serenity of trees and nature? If so, then you'll love the practice of mindful walking, also known as forest bathing. In this subchapter, we will explore how you can find joy in every step you take while immersing yourself in nature's embrace.

Mindful walking is a powerful practice that involves being fully present in the moment as you walk through a natural setting. It is a way to connect with the earth beneath your feet, the trees towering above you, and the sounds and smells of the forest that surround you. By slowing down and paying attention to each step you take, you can experience a sense of peace and tranquility that is hard to find in our fast-paced world.

As you practice mindful walking, you may find that your worries and stresses begin to melt away. The act of focusing on each step you take allows you to let go of the thoughts that are weighingyou down and instead focus on the beauty and wonder of the natural world around you. This can lead to a sense of calm and relaxation that can have a profound impact on your overall wellbeing.

In addition to the mental and emotional benefits of mindful walking, there are also physical benefits to be gained. Walking in nature has been shown to reduce stress, lower blood pressure, and improve mood. By incorporating mindful walking into your routine, you can experience these benefits while also connecting with the natural world in a deeper and more meaningful way.

So, if you're a nature lover looking to enhance your health and happiness, consider incorporating mindful walking into your daily routine. Take the time to slow down, breathe deeply, and connect with the beauty of the world around you. With each step you take, you can find joy, peace, and a sense of well-being that will leave you feeling rejuvenated and inspired.

Tree Hugging: Harnessing the Energy of Nature

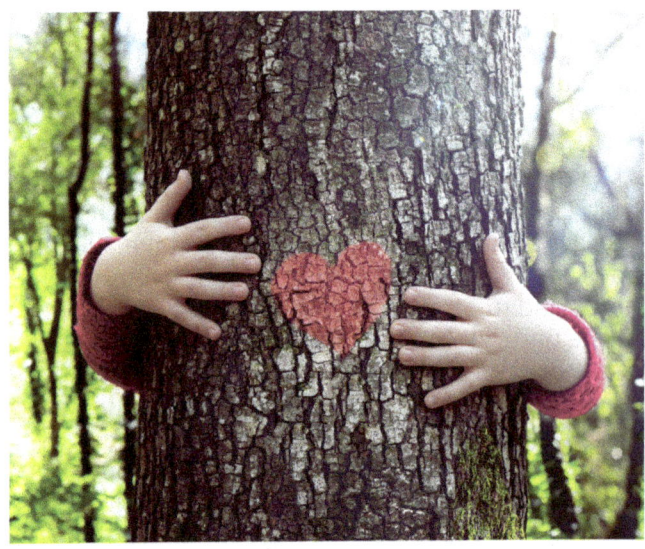

Welcome to the wonderful world of tree hugging! We will explore the incredible power of harnessing the energy of nature to promote health and happiness. For all you nature lovers, get ready to dive deep into the benefits of connecting with trees. Surrounding yourself with the beauty of the natural world.

Trees have long been revered for their ability to bring peace and tranquility to our lives. When we hug a tree, we are not only embracing a living being, but also tapping into its energy and vitality. Studies have shown that spending time in nature, particularly among trees, can reduce stress, anxiety, and depression. So next time you're feeling overwhelmed, take a moment to hug a tree and feel the calming effects wash over you.

The practice of tree hugging, also known as "forest bathing," has been gaining popularity as people seek ways to reconnect with nature and improve their overall well-being. By immersing ourselves in the natural world, we can experience a sense of grounding and renewal that is hard to find in our fast-paced, technology-driven lives. So go ahead, find a quiet spot in the forest, wrap your arms around a tree, and let its energy envelop you in a warm embrace.

Not only does tree hugging have mental health benefits, but it can also have a positive impact on our physical health. Trees release phytoncides, which are essential oils that have been shown to boost the immune system and reduce inflammation. Breathing in these healing compounds while hugging a tree can help strengthen your body's defenses and promote overall wellness. So the next time you feel a cold coming on, head to the nearest tree and give it a big hug for a natural immune boost.

In conclusion, tree hugging is not just a whimsical pastime for nature lovers – it is a powerful tool for enhancing our health and happiness. So whether you're feeling stressed, tired, or just in need of a little pick-me-up, take a moment to connect with the trees around you. Let their energy and vitality rejuvenate your mind, body, and spirit. Embrace the joy of forest bathing and experience the magic of nature's healing touch.

Nature Meditation: Quiet the Mind and Open the Heart

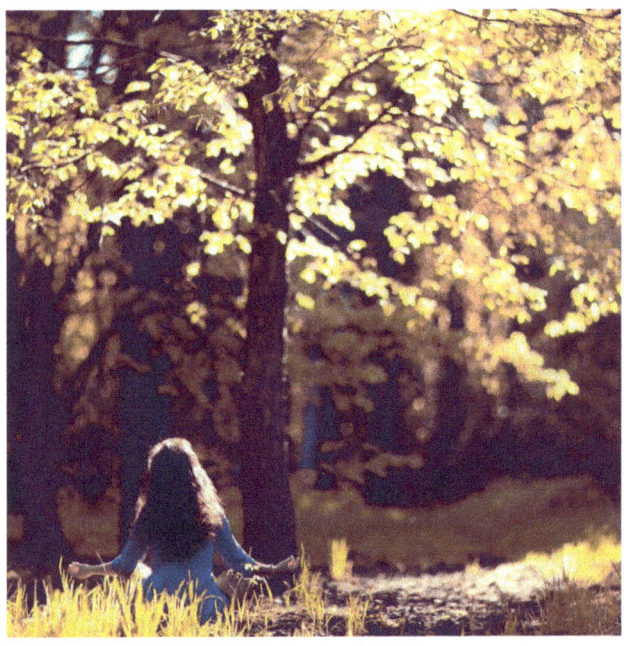

Nature meditation is a powerful practice that allows us to quiet the mind and open the heart to the beauty and energy of the natural world. For nature lovers, this form of meditation is a way to connect deeply with the earth and trees, finding peace and harmony in the midst of our busy lives.

By immersing ourselves in the sights, sounds, and smells of nature, we can tap into a sense of calm and serenity that is truly transformative.

When we take the time to sit quietly in nature, we allow ourselves to let go of the stresses and worries that often plague our minds. Instead, we focus on the present moment, tuning in to the rustling of leaves, the chirping of birds, and the gentle sway of the trees. This mindfulness practice helps us to release tension and anxiety, leaving us feeling refreshed and rejuvenated.

As we deepen our connection to nature through meditation, we begin to cultivate a sense of gratitude and appreciation for the natural world. We see the intricate beauty of a flower petal, the graceful dance of a butterfly, and the steadfast strength of a towering tree. This awareness of the interconnectedness of all living things fills our hearts with love and compassion, fostering a sense of unity and harmony with the world around us.

Through nature meditation, we not only find inner peace and healing, but we also experience a profound sense of joy and happiness. The simple act of being in nature, of breathing in the fresh air and feeling the sun on our skin, can lift our spirits and nourish our souls. We are reminded of the beauty and wonder of the world, inspiring us to live more fully and authentically.

So, to all the nature lovers out there, I encourage you to embrace the practice of naturemeditation. Allow yourself to be fully present in the natural world, to quiet your mind and open your heart to the healing power of trees and nature. In doing so, you will find a deep sense of joy and well-being that will carry you through even the most challenging of times.

Forest Breathing: Inhaling Fresh Air for Health and Happiness

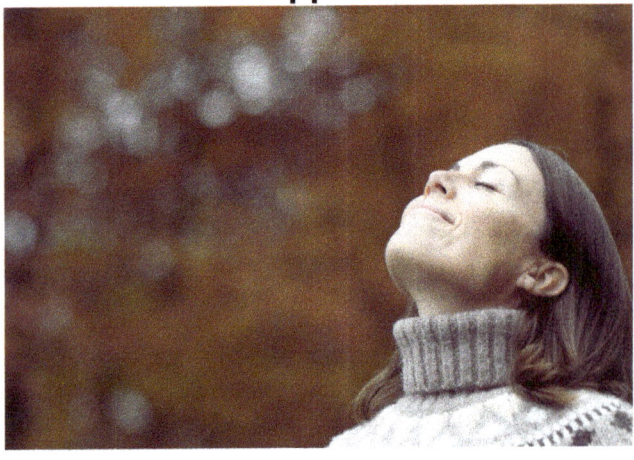

Step into the realm of forest breathing, where immersing yourself in the fresh, revitalizing air of verdant nature offers unmatched health and happiness. This section is crafted for nature enthusiasts, delving into the magic of connecting with the forest and discovering its profound healing powers.

Imagine taking a deep breath of crisp, clean forest air, filling your lungs with the pure essence of nature. This simple act of inhaling the fresh air around trees has been shown to have numerous health benefits, from reducing stress and anxiety to boosting the immune system and improving overall well-being. The forest truly is a natural pharmacy, offering us the gift of clean, oxygenrich air to breathe in deeply.

Studies have shown that spending time in nature, particularly among trees, can have a profound impact on our mental and physical health. The Japanese practice of Shinrin Yoku, or forest bathing, emphasizes the importance of immersing oneself in the sights, sounds, and scents of the forest to promote relaxation and stress relief. By simply taking a leisurely stroll through the woods and inhaling the fresh forest air, we can experience a sense of calm and rejuvenation that is hard to find elsewhere.

The act of forest breathing is not just about inhaling oxygen; it is about connecting with the natural world and allowing ourselves to be fully present in the moment. As we breathe in the fresh air and take in the beauty of the forest around us, we can feel a sense of awe and wonder that fills us with joy and gratitude. The healing powers of nature are truly remarkable, and by spending time in the forest and breathing in its fresh air, we can tap into a source of health and happiness that is always available to us.

Nature lovers out there, remember to take the time to immerse yourself in the beauty of the forest and inhale its fresh air deeply. Allow yourself to be present in the moment and let the healing powers of nature work their magic on your mind, body, and soul. Embrace the joy of forest bathing and let the trees surround you with their

love and support as you breathe

in the gift of fresh air for health and happiness.

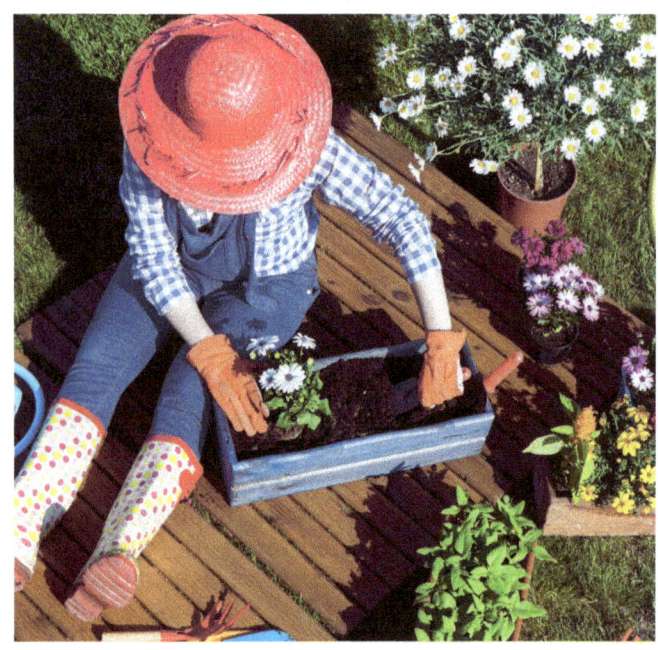

Chapter 4: Creating Your Own Nature Sanctuary

Designing a Sacred Space in Your Backyard

Are you a nature lover looking to create a sacred space in your backyard where you can connect with the healing power of trees and nature? Look no further! In this subchapter of "The Joy of Forest Bathing: Embracing Nature for Health and Happiness," we will explore how you can design a sacred space in your very own backyard that will bring you joy and wellness.

The first step in designing a sacred space in your backyard is to choose a location that is tranquil and peaceful. Look for a spot that is surrounded by trees, plants, and other elements of nature that will help you feel connected to the earth. Consider creating a seating area where you can sit and meditate, read, or simply enjoy the beauty of your surroundings.

Next, think about incorporating elements of nature into your sacred space. Plant native trees, shrubs, and flowers that will attract birds, butterflies, and other wildlife. Consider adding a water feature, such as a small pond or fountain, to create a soothing atmosphere. You may also want to include natural materials, such as rocks, stones, and wood, to enhance the natural feel of your space.

In addition to incorporating elements of nature into your sacred space, consider adding personal touches that reflect your own spiritual beliefs and practices. You could create a small altar with candles, crystals, or other sacred objects that are meaningful to you. You may also want to hang wind chimes, prayer flags, or other decorations that will enhance the spiritual energy of your space.

Finally, don't forget to take care of your sacred space by regularly tending to the plants, trees, and other elements that make it special. Spend time in your sacred space each day, whether it's for meditation, yoga, or simply enjoying the beauty of nature. By creating a sacred space in your backyard, you will not only enhance your connection to nature but also experience greater

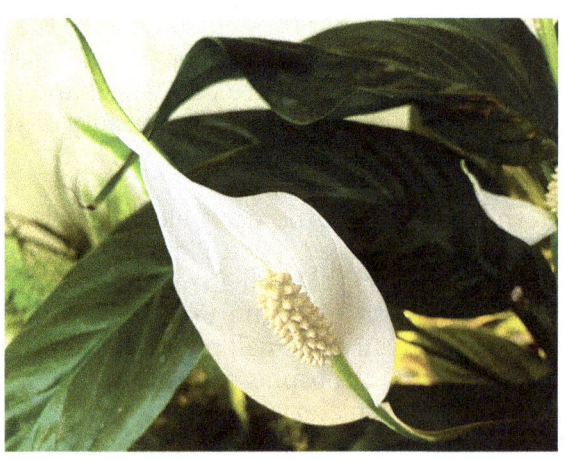

health and happiness in your life.

Bringing the Outdoors Inside: Houseplants for Health

Are you a nature lover looking to bring the outdoors inside? Look no further than houseplants! In this subchapter, we will explore the benefits of incorporating houseplants into your home for both your health and happiness. Houseplants not only add beauty and life to your living space, but they can also improve air quality, reduce stress, and boost overall well-being.

Houseplants have been shown to have a positive impact on our health by purifying the air in our homes. Plants such as spider plants, pothos, and peace lilies are known for their ability to remove toxins like formaldehyde, benzene, and trichloroethylene from the air. By adding these plants to your indoor environment, you can breathe easier and enjoy cleaner, fresher air.

In addition to their air-purifying properties, houseplants can also help to reduce stress and improve mental health. Studies have shown that being around plants can lower blood pressure, reduce anxiety, and promote relaxation. The presence of greenery in your home can create a calming and peaceful atmosphere, making it the perfect retreat from the hustle and bustle of daily life.

Not only do houseplants benefit our physical and mental health, but they also have a positive impact on our overall well-being. Caring for plants can provide a sense of purpose and accomplishment, as well as a connection to nature. Watching your plants grow and thrive can bring a sense of joy and satisfaction, fostering a deeper appreciation for the natural world.

So, whether you're a seasoned plant enthusiast or looking to green up your space for the first time, houseplants are a fantastic way to bring the outdoors inside and reap the many health benefits they have to offer. Embrace the joy of surrounding

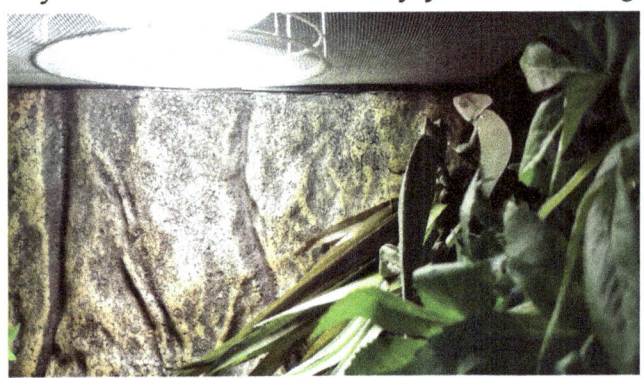

yourself with nature and trees in the comfort of your own home, and watch as your happiness and well-being flourish.

Nature-Inspired Crafts and DIY Projects

Nature lovers rejoice! In this subchapter, we will

explore the world of nature-inspired crafts and DIY projects that will bring the beauty of the outdoors into your home. Whether you are looking to add a touch of nature to your living space or simply want to immerse yourself in the calming and healing powers of the natural world, these projects are sure to inspire and delight.

One of the simplest ways to incorporate nature into your home is by creating your own botanical art. Gather leaves, flowers, and other natural materials from your surroundings and press them between the pages of a heavy book to preserve their beauty. Once dried, arrange them in a frame or shadow box to create a stunning piece of art that will remind you of the tranquility of the forest every time you gaze upon it.

For those with a green thumb, why not try your hand at creating a terrarium? These miniature ecosystems are not only beautiful to look at but also provide a sense of peace and tranquility. Gather moss, small plants, and pebbles from the forest floor and arrange them in a glass container to create your own little slice of nature. Place your terrarium in a sunny spot in your home and watch as it thrives and brings a touch of the outdoors indoors.

If you are feeling crafty, consider making your own natural candles using beeswax and essential oils. Not only are these candles environmentally friendly, but they also emit a soothing and calming fragrance that will transport you to a peaceful forest glade. Experiment with different scents such as pine, lavender, or eucalyptus to find the perfect aroma that will help you relax and unwind after a long day.

Finally, why not take your love of nature a step further by creating your own herbal remedies and skincare products? Gather herbs such as lavender, chamomile, and mint from your garden or local forest and infuse them into oils, balms, and salves. Not only will these homemade products nourish your skin and body, but they will also connect you to the healing powers of the natural world in a deeply meaningful way. Gather your supplies, and let nature inspire you to create beauty and wellness in your own home.

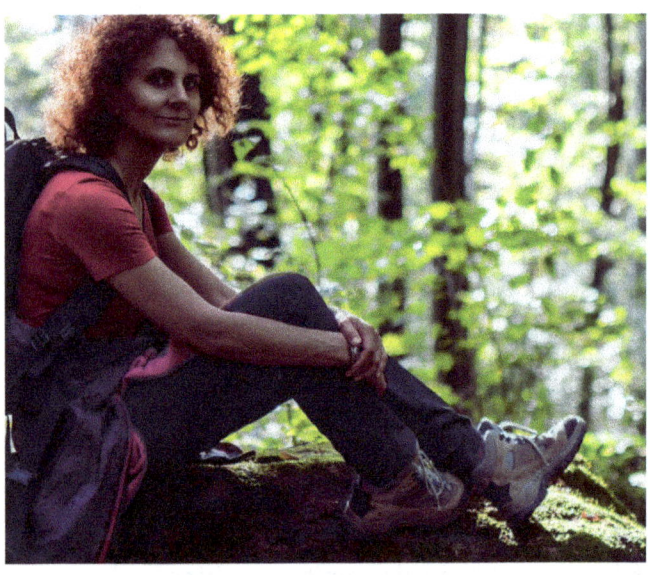

Planning a Nature Retreat: Connecting with the Wild

Are you a nature lover looking to take your appreciation for the great outdoors to the next level? Look no further than planning a nature retreat to connect with the wild and experience the healing powers of nature firsthand! In this subchapter, we will explore the benefits of immersing yourself in the natural world, how to plan the perfect nature retreat, and tips for making the most of your time in the wild.

Nature has a way of rejuvenating the mind, body, and soul like nothing else can. From the calming sounds of a babbling brook to the fresh scent of pine trees, spending time in nature has been scientifically proven to reduce stress, boost mood, and improve overall well-being. By planning a nature retreat, you can fully immerse yourself in the healing powers of the natural world and reap the benefits of forest bathing for yourself.

When planning a nature retreat, consider the type of environment you want to immerse yourself in. Do you prefer the tranquility of a secluded forest, the rugged beauty of a mountain landscape, or the soothing sounds of the ocean? Choose a location that speaks to your soul and allows you to fully connect with the wild. Research different nature retreat options, from camping in a national park to booking a cabin in the woods, and find the perfect setting for your rejuvenating getaway.

Once you have chosen your ideal location, it's time to plan your nature retreat itinerary. Consider activities such as hiking, birdwatching, meditation, or simply sitting quietly and soaking in the sights and sounds of nature. Make time for self-reflection, journaling, and connecting with the natural world around you. Remember, the goal of a nature retreat is to slow down, disconnect from the hustle and bustle of daily life, and fully embrace the healing powers of the wild.

As you embark on your nature retreat, remember to stay present in the moment and open yourself up to the beauty and wonder of the natural world. Take deep breaths, listen to the sounds of nature, and allow yourself to be fully immersed in the healing energy of the wild. By connecting with nature on a deeper level, you can experience true happiness and find peace and tranquility in the beauty of the natural world. So pack your bags, lace up your hiking boots, and get ready to embark on a nature retreat like no other!

Chapter 5: Embracing the Seasons

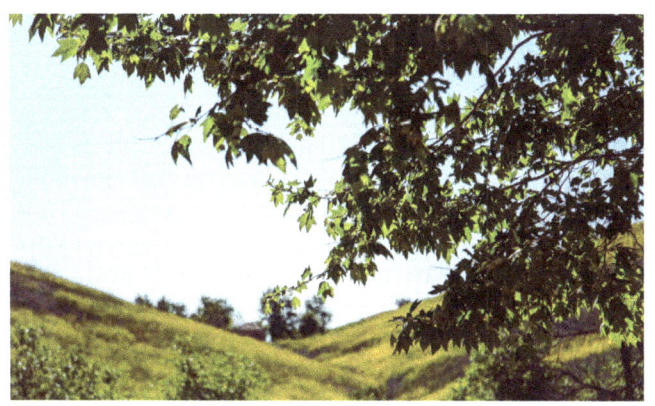

Spring Renewal: Awakening Your Senses

Welcome to the subchapter on "Spring Renewal: Awakening Your Senses" in our book, "The Joy of Forest Bathing: Embracing Nature for Health and Happiness." For all you nature lovers out there, this is the perfect time to reconnect with the beauty and magic of the natural world as spring brings new life and energy to the forests. In this subchapter, we will explore how immersing yourself in nature during the spring season can awaken your senses and bring about a sense of renewal and rejuvenation.

As the winter chill fades away, the vibrant colors and fragrances of blooming flowers and fresh green leaves fill the air, stimulating our sense of sight and smell. Take a moment to breathe in the sweet scent of blossoms and listen to the symphony of birdsong as you walk through the forest. Notice how the colors of spring awaken your visual senses, filling you with a sense of wonder and awe at the beauty of the natural world.

Spring is a time of rebirth and growth, and immersing yourself in nature during this season can help you tap into that energy of renewal. Take off your shoes and feel the soft earth beneath your feet, connecting with the earth's energy and grounding yourself in the present moment. Let the warmth of the sun on your skin and the gentle breeze on your face awaken your sense of touch, bringing you a sense of peace and harmony with the natural world.

Incorporating mindfulness practices such as deep breathing, meditation, and yoga into your forest bathing experience can help you fully engage your senses and deepen your connection with nature. As you focus on your breath and quiet your mind, you may find yourself more attuned to the sights, sounds, and sensations of the forest around you. Allow yourself to be fully present in the moment, embracing the beauty and wonder of the natural world with an open heart and mind.

Nature lovers, as you venture into the forest this spring, remember to awaken your senses and embrace the renewal and rejuvenation that nature has to offer. Let the sights, sounds, and sensations of the natural world fill you with joy and gratitude, and allow yourself to be fully immersed in the healing energy of the forest. May your spring forest bathing experiences bring you health, happiness, and a deep sense of connection with the beauty of the world around you.

Summer Bliss: Basking in the Warmth of the Sun

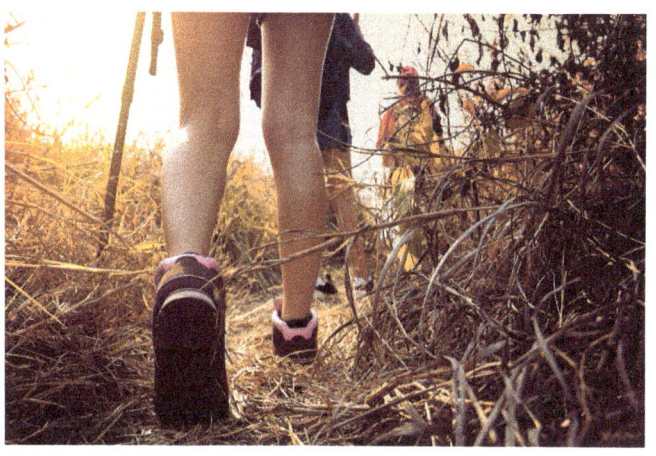

Ah, summer! The season of sunshine, warmth, and endless possibilities. There is no better time to immerse ourselves in the great outdoors and soak up the healing powers of the sun. As we step outside and feel the rays on our skin, we can't help but feel a sense of joy and contentment wash over us. The sun's warmth is not just a physical sensation, but a spiritual one as well, connecting us to the natural world in a profound way.

Basking in the warmth of the sun is a time-honored tradition that has been practiced for centuries. From ancient civilizations to modern-day wellness enthusiasts, people have recognized the incredible benefits of sunlight on both the body and the mind. The sun's rays provide us with much-needed vitamin D, which is essential for strong bones, a healthy immune system, and overall well-being. But beyond the physical benefits, there is something truly magical about sitting in the sun and feeling its energy flow through us, revitalizing and rejuvenating our spirits.

As we embrace the summer months and spend more time outdoors, we have the opportunity to truly connect with nature and all its wonders. Whether we are lounging in a hammock under a canopy of trees, hiking through a sun-dappled forest, or picnicking in a lush meadow, we are surrounded by the beauty and abundance of the natural world. The sun's warm embrace only enhances this experience, filling us with a sense of gratitude and awe for the world around us.

In a world that is often fast-paced and stressful, taking the time to bask in the warmth of the sun can be a powerful antidote to the pressures of daily life. As we slow down, breathe deeply, and let the sun's rays wash over us, we can feel our worries melt away and our hearts fill with joy. The practice of sun basking is a simple yet profound way to reconnect with ourselves and the world around us, reminding us of the healing power of nature and the importance of taking time to nurture our bodies and souls.

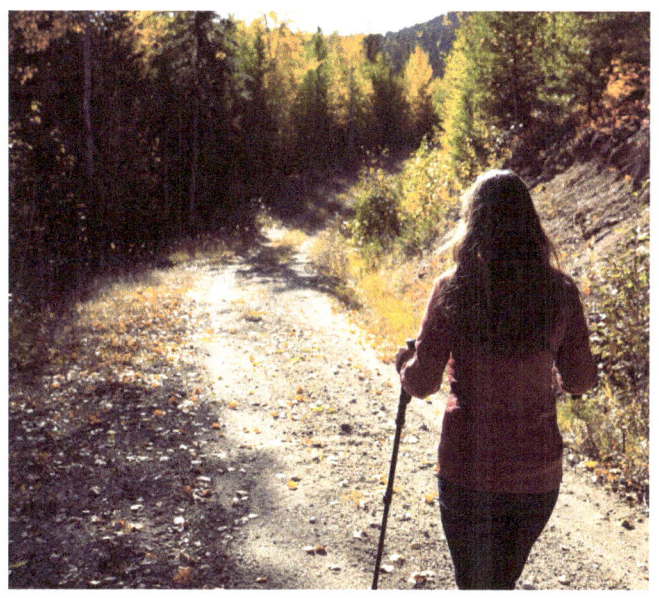

Let us embrace the summer bliss and bask in the warmth of the sun. Let us revel in the beauty of the natural world and all its wonders. And let us remember that in the simple act of sitting in the sun, we can find happiness, health, and a deep sense of connection to the world around us.

Fall Harvest: Celebrating the Bounty of Nature

As the leaves begin to change colors and the air turns crisp, the fall season brings with it a sense of abundance and gratitude for the bountiful harvest that nature provides. For nature lovers, this is a time to celebrate the beauty and abundance of the natural world, and to immerse ourselves in the wonders of the forest.

Fall harvest is a time to reap the rewards of the hard work and dedication of farmers andgardeners, as well as to appreciate the gifts that nature bestows upon us. From the vibrant hues of pumpkins and squash to the sweet flavors of ripe apples and pears, the fall harvest is a feast for the senses that nourishes both body and soul.

For those who practice forest bathing, the fall harvest season offers a unique opportunity toconnect with nature in a deeper and more meaningful way. The changing colors of the leaves, the crispness of the air, and the abundance of fruits and vegetables all contribute to a sense of renewal and rejuvenation that can only be found in the forest.

As we take in the sights, sounds, and smells of the fall harvest season, we are reminded of theinterconnectedness of all living things and the importance of honoring and respecting the natural world. By celebrating the bounty of nature, we not only nourish our bodies with fresh, seasonal foods, but we also nourish our souls with a sense of wonder and awe at the beauty and abundance that surrounds us.

So as we embrace the fall harvest season, let us take the time to slow down, breathe deeply, and immerse ourselves in the healing power of nature.

Let us give thanks for the bountiful gifts that the earth provides, and let us revel in the joy and happiness that comes from connecting with the natural world.

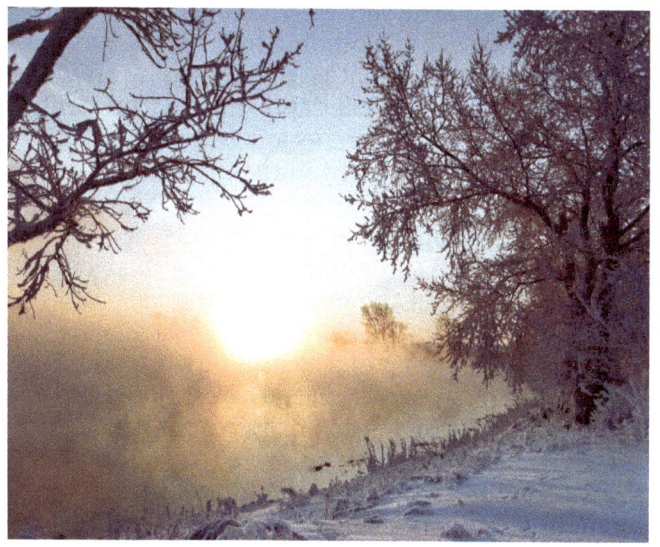

Winter Reflection: Finding Peace in Stillness

Winter is a time of quiet contemplation and reflection, when the world slows down and nature takes a much-needed rest. For those of us who love spending time in the great outdoors, this season offers a unique opportunity to find peace in the stillness of the forest. As the trees stand bare and silent, their branches reaching up to the sky like outstretched arms, we can't help but be reminded of the beauty and resilience of nature.

There is something truly magical about the way the winter landscape transforms the forest into a serene and tranquil sanctuary. The crunch of snow beneath our boots, the crisp bite of the cold air on our cheeks, and the soft whisper of the wind through the trees all combine to create a sense of peace and harmony that is unmatched by any other season. In this quiet and still environment, we can let go of the stresses and worries of daily life and simply be present in the moment.

As we immerse ourselves in the beauty of the winter forest, we can't help but feel a sense of wonder and awe at the majesty of the natural world. The stark beauty of the bare branches against the backdrop of a clear blue sky, the delicate tracery of frost on the forest floor, and the occasional flash of a deer or squirrel darting through the underbrush all serve to remind us of the interconnectedness of all living things. In this moment of stillness, we can feel a deep sense of gratitude for the beauty and abundance that surrounds us.

In the stillness of the winter forest, we have the opportunity to connect with our inner selves and find a sense of peace and tranquility that is often elusive in our busy modern lives. As we walk among the trees, breathing in the crisp, clean air and feeling the warmth of the winter sun on our faces, we can't help but feel a sense of renewal and rejuvenation. The forest offers us a space to let go of our worries and fears, to quiet our minds and open our hearts to the beauty and wonder of the natural world.

So, to all the nature lovers out there, I encourage you to embrace the magic of the winter forest and find peace in its stillness. Take a moment to step outside, breathe in the fresh air, and let the beauty of the trees and the tranquility of the forest wash over you. In this moment of connection with nature, you will find not only happiness and health, but a deep sense of peace and contentment that will stay with you long after you have left the forest behind.

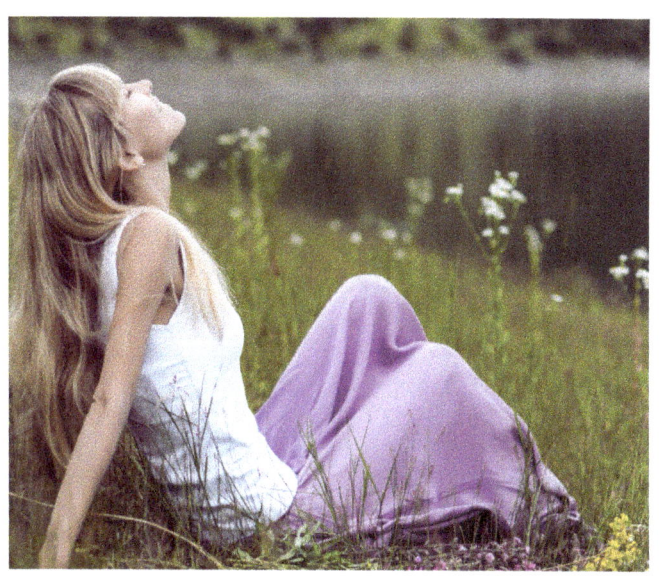

Chapter 6: The Joy of Forest Bathing for Health and Happiness

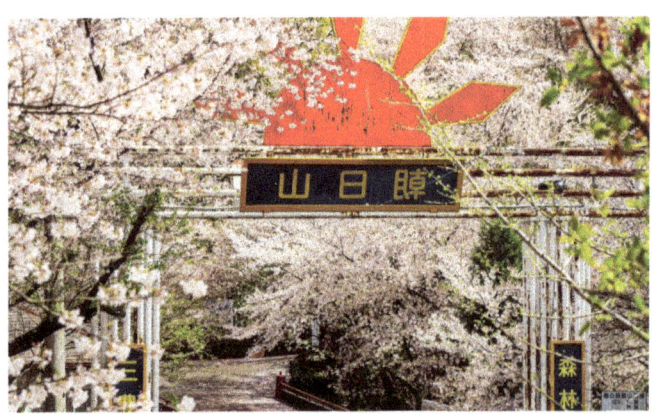

Healing the Body, Mind, and Spirit with Nature

Are you a nature lover looking to enhance your health and happiness? Then you're in for a treat with this subchapter on "Healing the Body, Mind, and Spirit with Nature" from our book, "The Joy of Forest Bathing: Embracing Nature for Health and Happiness." We believe that connecting with nature is the key to unlocking a world of healing for your body, mind, and spirit.

Nature has a way of working its magic on us, rejuvenating our bodies, calming our minds, and uplifting our spirits. When we immerse ourselves in the natural world, whether it's by taking a leisurely walk through a forest or simply sitting under a tree, we allow ourselves to be enveloped in the healing energies of nature. The fresh air, the gentle rustling of leaves, and the vibrant colors of the flora all work together to create a sense of peace and well-being within us.

Studies have shown that spending time in nature can have numerous health benefits, including reducing stress, lowering blood pressure, and boosting our immune systems. The practice of forest bathing, which involves immersing oneself in the sights, sounds, and smells of the forest, has been shown to have profound effects on our overall well-being. By simply being present in nature and allowing ourselves to connect with the trees and plants around us, we can experience a sense of calm and rejuvenation that can't be found anywhere else.

The Japanese Practice of Shinrin-Yoku

Shinrin-yoku, which translates to "forest bathing" or "taking in the forest atmosphere," is a Japanese practice that encourages people to immerse themselves in nature to enhance theirwell-being. Originating in Japan in the 1980s, shinrin-yoku was developed as a response to the increasing levels of stress and burnout associated with urbanization and a fast-paced lifestyle. It is now a cornerstone of preventive health care and healing in Japanese medicine.

The Philosophy Behind Shinrin-Yoku

At its core, shinrin-yoku is about slowing down and experiencing nature with all your senses. It's not about hiking or exercising vigorously; instead, it's about being mindful and present in the natural environment. This practice encourages people to:

- See the beauty of the natural surroundings, from the vastness of the forest to the intricatedetails of leaves and flowers.

- Hear the sounds of the forest, such as the rustling of leaves, bird songs, and the gentle flow of streams.

- Smell the fresh, earthy scents of the woods, which can be particularly invigorating.

- Touch the textures of trees, plants, and the forest floor.

- Taste the clean, crisp air and sometimes even wild edibles under guidance.

Health Benefits of Shinrin-Yoku

Numerous scientific studies have documented the health benefits of shinrin-yoku, highlighting its profound impact on both physical and mental health:

- Stress Reduction: Shinrin-yoku has been shown to lower levels of cortisol, the stress hormone, thereby reducing stress and anxiety.

- Enhanced Immune Function: Spending time in the forest can increase the activity and number of natural killer (NK) cells, which play a crucial role in the immune system's defense against infections and cancer.

- Improved Mood: Forest bathing can lead to a significant decrease in symptoms of depression and anxiety, promoting a more positive mood.

- Lower Blood Pressure: Regular exposure to forest environments can help lower blood pressure, reducing the risk of heart disease.

- Increased Energy: Participants often report feeling more energetic and less fatigued after spending time in the forest.

- Better Sleep: Exposure to natural light and the calming effects of nature can improve sleep quality.

How to Practice Shinrin-Yoku

To practice shinrin-yoku, you don't need special equipment or extensive planning. Here are some simple steps to get started:

1. Find a Forest or Natural Area: Choose a place that feels welcoming and safe. It doesn't have to be a large forest; even a small park can offer benefits.

2. Unplug: Leave your phone and other distractions behind to fully engage with your surroundings.

3. Walk Slowly: Take your time to wander aimlessly and let your senses guide you. There's no destination or goal other than to be present.

4. Engage Your Senses: Pay attention to what you see, hear, smell, and feel. Sit down, if you like, and simply observe.

5. Breathe Deeply: Practice deep breathing to help relax and center your mind.

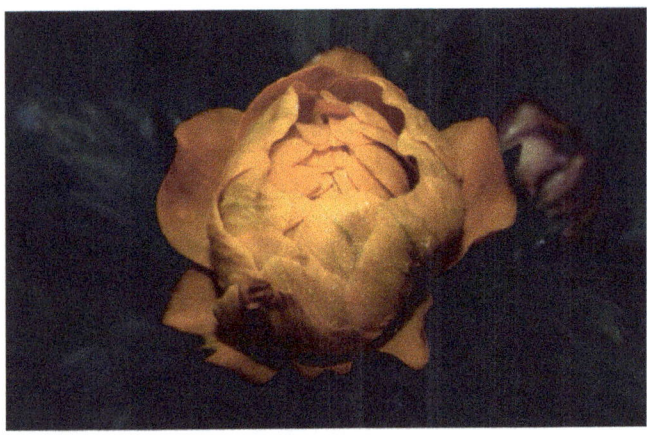

6. Stay for a While: Aim to spend at least 20-30 minutes in the forest, though longer sessions of two hours or more can provide even greater benefits.

Shinrin-yoku is a simple yet powerful way to reconnect with nature and yourself. By incorporating this practice into your life, you can tap into the healing powers of the natural world and cultivate a greater sense of peace and well-being.

But the healing power of nature goes beyond just the physical benefits. Connecting with nature also has a profound impact on our mental and emotional well-being. Being surrounded by the beauty and serenity of the natural world can help to clear our minds, reduce anxiety, and increase our sense of gratitude and appreciation for life. It's no wonder that so many people turn to nature as a source of comfort and solace during difficult times.

So, if you're looking to enhance your health and happiness, we encourage you to embrace the healing power of nature. Whether it's taking a leisurely stroll through a park, spending time in a garden, or simply sitting under a tree, make time to connect with the natural world around you. Your body, mind, and spirit will thank you for it, and you'll find yourself feeling happier and healthier than ever before. Embrace the joy of forest bathing and let nature work its magic on you!

Cultivating Gratitude for the Gifts of the Earth

As nature lovers, we are constantly in awe of the

gifts that the Earth provides us with, especially the healing and rejuvenating power of trees. In this subchapter, we will explore the importance of cultivating gratitude for the gifts of the Earth, particularly in the form of forest bathing. This practice allows us to connect with nature on a deeper level and experience the health and happiness that comes from immersing ourselves in the beauty of the natural world.

When we take the time to slow down and appreciate the trees around us, we open ourselves up to a world of healing and joy. Trees have a way of grounding us, of reminding us of our place in the natural order of things. By cultivating gratitude for the gifts of the Earth, we can tap into the energy and wisdom that trees have to offer, allowing us to feel more at peace and in tune with the world around us.

One of the simplest ways to cultivate gratitude for the gifts of the Earth is to spend time in nature, whether it's by taking a leisurely walk through the forest or simply sitting under a tree and soaking in its energy. By immersing ourselves in the sights, sounds, and scents of the natural world, we can connect with the Earth in a way that is both healing and transformative. This connection can bring us a sense of peace and contentment that is hard to find anywhere else.

In addition to spending time in nature, we can also cultivate gratitude for the gifts of the Earth by practicing mindfulness and gratitude exercises. By taking the time to notice and appreciate the beauty and abundance that surrounds us, we can shift our focus from what we lack to what we have, fostering a sense of gratitude and contentment that can have a profound impact on our overall well-being. This practice can help us to feel more connected to the Earth and more appreciative of the gifts that it provides us with.

In conclusion, cultivating gratitude for the gifts of the Earth is essential for anyone who wants to experience the full benefits of forest bathing and connect with the healing power of nature. By taking the time to appreciate the beauty and abundance that surrounds us, we can tap into the energy and wisdom of the natural world, allowing us to feel more at peace and in tune with the Earth. So, let us embrace the practice of gratitude and open ourselves up to the wonders of the natural world, for there is much joy and healing to be found in the gifts of the Earth.

Finding Joy in the Simple Pleasures of Nature Are you a nature lover who finds joy and peace in the simple pleasures of the great outdoors? If so, you are in for a treat with the practice of forest bathing. In this subchapter, we will explore how immersing yourself in nature can bring happiness and healing to your mind, body, and soul.

One of the greatest joys of spending time in nature is the ability to connect with the beauty and wonder of the natural world. Whether it's the sight of towering trees reaching towards the sky, the sound of birds chirping in the distance, or the feel of cool earth beneath your feet, every moment spent in nature is a moment of pure bliss. By taking the time to appreciate these simple pleasures, you can experience a profound sense of joy and gratitude for the world around you.

In addition to the emotional benefits of connecting with nature, spending time outdoors has been shown to have numerous health benefits as well. From reducing stress and anxiety to boosting immunity and improving overall well-being, the healing power of nature is truly remarkable. By embracing the simple pleasures of nature through activities like forest bathing, you can experience a renewed sense of vitality and energy that will carry over into all aspects of your life.

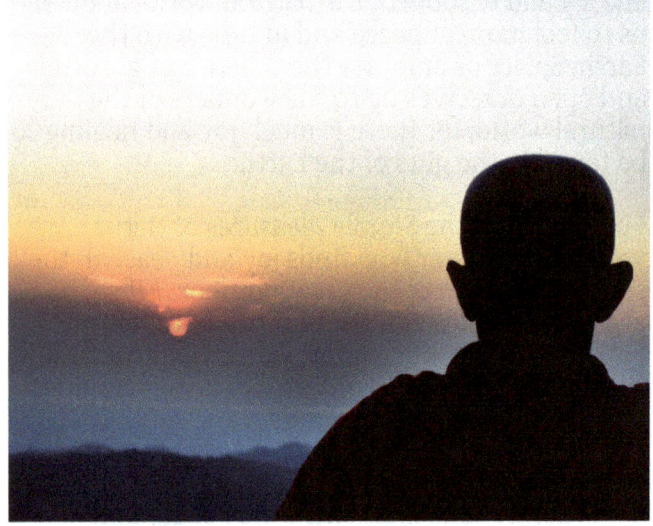

As a nature lover, you understand the importance of preserving and protecting the natural world for future generations to enjoy. By finding joy in the simple pleasures of nature, you can cultivate a deep appreciation for the beauty and diversity of the world around you. Whether you are hiking through a lush forest, picnicking in a sunny meadow, or simply sitting under a shady tree, take the time to savor each moment and let the healing power of nature wash over you.

So, fellow nature lovers, let us embrace the simple pleasures of nature and bask in the joy and healing that it brings. Whether you are seeking happiness, health, or simply a sense of peace and tranquility, spending time in nature is sure to bring a smile to your face and a warmth to your heart. So go ahead, step outside, take a deep breath, and let the beauty of the natural world surround you.

Embracing the Wisdom of the Forest: Lessons in Resilience and Growth

Step into the forest and feel the magic of nature enveloping you, inviting you to slow down and embrace its wisdom. In the hustle and bustle of our daily lives, we often forget to connect with the natural world around us. But when we take the time to immerse ourselves in the serene beauty of the forest, we are rewarded with valuable lessons in resilience and growth.

The forest is a living, breathing ecosystem that has weathered countless storms and hallenges over the centuries. From towering trees that have stood the test of time to delicate ferns that thrive in the shade, each plant and animal in the forest has its own story of resilience to share. By observing and learning from the remarkable ability of nature to adapt and flourish in the face of adversity, we can gain valuable insights into our own capacity for growth and strength.

Just as the forest teaches us resilience, it also reminds us of the importance of growth. Trees start as tiny seeds and grow into majestic beings that provide shelter and sustenance for countless creatures. In the same way, we too have the potential to grow and evolve, overcoming obstacles and reaching new heights in our personal and professional lives. The forest serves as a powerful reminder that growth is a natural and essential part of life, and that by embracing change and challenges, we can become our best selves.

As nature lovers, we are drawn to the healing powers of trees and the forest. Studies have shown that spending time in nature can lower stress

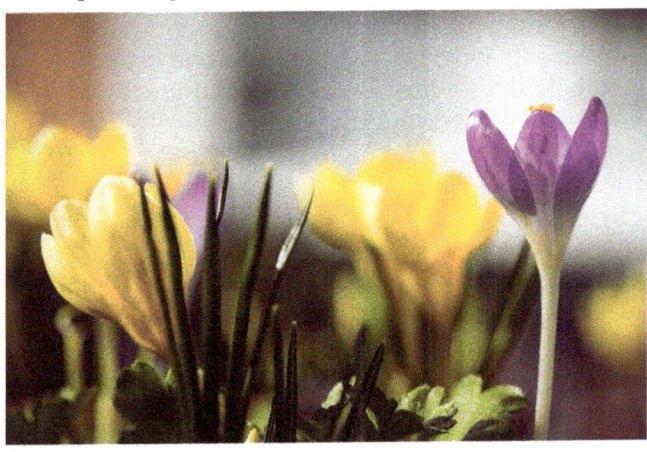

levels, improve mood, and boost overall well-being. Forest bathing, or immersing oneself in the sights, sounds, and scents of the forest, has been proven to have numerous health benefits, from reducing blood pressure to enhancing immune function. By embracing the wisdom of the forest and allowing ourselves to be fully present in its beauty, we can experience a profound sense of peace and rejuvenation.

So, let us take a moment to step away from our screens and responsibilities, and venture into the welcoming embrace of the forest. Let us open our hearts and minds to the lessons of resilience and growth that nature has to offer, and allow ourselves to be nourished and inspired by the wisdom of the trees. In doing so, we can cultivate a deeper connection to the natural world and find true happiness and health in its tranquil embrace.

Conclusion: Living a Life in Harmony with Nature

In conclusion, living a life in harmony with nature is the key to finding true happiness and health. As nature lovers, we already understand the profound benefits that come from immersing ourselves in the beauty of the natural world. Whether it's taking a leisurely stroll through a lush forest, breathing in the fresh air of a meadow, or simply sitting under the shade of a mighty oak tree, connecting with nature is essential for our overall well-being.

By embracing the practice of forest bathing, we can truly tap into the healing powers of nature. Research has shown that spending time in forests can reduce stress, lower blood pressure, and boost our immune system. The simple act of being surrounded by trees and listening to the sounds of nature can have a profound impact on our mental and physical health. It is a powerful reminder of the interconnectedness of all living things and the importance of taking care of our planet.

As we continue to prioritize our relationship with nature, we are not only benefiting ourselves but also the environment around us. By respecting and cherishing the natural world, we are contributing to the preservation of our planet for future generations. Our love for nature fuels our desire to protect it, leading to a more sustainable and harmonious existence for all living beings.

So let us continue to seek out moments of tranquility in nature, to revel in the beauty of our surroundings, and to cultivate a deep appreciation for the wonders of the natural world. By living a life in harmony with nature, we are not only nurturing our own well-being but also fostering a sense of peace and balance in our lives. Let us celebrate the joy of forest bathing and embrace the healing power of nature for health and happiness.

Acknowledgments

In writing this book, "The Joy of Forest Bathing: Embracing Nature for Health and Happiness," I am overwhelmed with gratitude for the incredible support and inspiration that has fueled this project. To all the nature lovers out there, this book is dedicated to you - those who understand the healing power of trees and the beauty of the great outdoors. Your passion for nature has ignited a fire within me to share the wonders of forest bathing with the world.

I would like to express my deepest appreciation to all the experts, researchers, and practitioners in the field of forest bathing who have generously shared their knowledge and insights with me. Without their expertise and dedication, this book would not have been possible. Their passion for promoting health and happiness through nature is truly inspiring, and I am honored to have had the opportunity to learn from them.

I also want to extend my heartfelt thanks to all the trees and forests that have provided a sanctuary for me to connect with nature and find peace and tranquility. The wisdom and beauty of the natural world have been a constant source of joy and inspiration in my life, and I am forever grateful for the healing power of trees.

To my readers, I am grateful for your curiosity and openness to exploring the benefits of forest bathing. Your willingness to embrace nature as a source of health and happiness is a testament to the transformative power of the great outdoors. I hope that this book will inspire you to connect with nature in new and meaningful ways, and that you will find joy and healing in the beauty of the natural world.

In closing, I want to express my deepest gratitude to all those who have supported me on this journey - family, friends, colleagues, and readers alike. Your belief in the importance of nature for health and happiness has been a constant source of encouragement and inspiration. Together, let us continue to embrace the joy of forest bathing and celebrate the wonders of the natural world. Thank you from the bottom of my heart.

Resources for Further Exploration

Are you a nature lover who can't get enough of the healing powers of the great outdoors? If so, you're in luck! In this subchapter, we will explore some fantastic resources for further exploration of the benefits of forest bathing and connecting with nature. Whether you're looking to deepen your understanding of the science behind the healing effects of nature or simply seeking more ways to incorporate nature into your daily life, these resources will inspire and uplift you on your journey to health and happiness.

For those interested in delving deeper into the research and science behind the benefits of spending time in nature, there are several books and articles that provide in-depth explanations of how nature can improve our mental and physical well-being. "The Nature Fix" by Florence Williams is a must-read for anyone curious about the science of nature therapy, while articles from publications such as National Geographic and The New York Times offer fascinating insights into the latest research on the subject.

If you're looking for practical tips on how to incorporate more nature into your daily life, there are a wealth of resources available to help you do just that. Websites such as Forest Therapy Hub and The Nature Fix offer advice on everything from creating a nature-inspired home to planning a forest bathing retreat. Additionally, social media platforms like Instagram and Pinterest are filled with accounts dedicated to sharing beautiful images of nature and inspiring quotes about the healing powers of the natural world.

For those seeking a more immersive experience in nature, there are countless organizations and retreat centers that offer guided forest bathing walks and nature-based workshops. The Association of Nature and Forest Therapy Guides and Programs provides a directory of certified guides who can lead you on a transformative journey through the forest, while retreat centers like The Esalen Institute and 1440 Multiversity offer weekend workshops and immersive experiences in nature that will leave you feeling rejuvenated and inspired.

Whether you're a seasoned nature lover or just beginning to explore the benefits of connecting with the natural world, these resources are sure to provide you with the inspiration and information you need to deepen your relationship with nature and experience the profound healing and happiness that can come from spending time among the trees. So go ahead, dive in, and let the magic of the forest envelop you in its embrace. Your mind, body, and spirit will thank you for it!

About the Author

Are you a nature lover who can't get enough of the great outdoors and the healing power of trees? Then you're in for a treat with "The Joy of Forest Bathing: Embracing Nature for Health and Happiness"! Let me introduce myself - I am the author of this book, a dedicated nature enthusiast who has spent years studying the benefits of immersing oneself in the beauty of the natural world.

My passion for nature and its ability to heal and rejuvenate our minds, bodies, and souls is what inspired me to write this book. I truly believe that spending time in nature, especially among trees, can have a profound impact on our overall well-being. From reducing stress and anxiety to boosting our immune system and increasing our energy levels, the benefits of forest bathing are endless.

In "The Joy of Forest Bathing," I share my personal experiences with nature and how it has transformed my life for the better. I delve into the science behind the healing powers of trees and provide practical tips and techniques for incorporating forest bathing into your daily routine. Whether you're looking to improve your mental health, strengthen your physical body, or simply find more joy and happiness in your life, this book has something for everyone.

Join me on a journey of discovery as we explore the wonders of nature and the magic of forest bathing together. Let's embrace the healing power of trees and unlock the secrets to a happier, healthier life. Get ready to immerse yourself in the beauty of the natural world and experience the joy and wonder that comes from connecting with the great outdoors.

www.ingramcontent.com/pod-product-compliance
Lightning Source LLC
Chambersburg PA
CBHW070518090426
42735CB00012B/2833